In All Things

MODERATION

One Woman's Answer to the Question: How do you stay so thin?

5 Common Sense Steps to a New Way of Eating

ELIZABETH STEVENSON

FOR KEIFER

CHAPTER 1

"How do you stay so thin?" I asked her. And I remember we were sitting in her office and she was eating...I don't know, I think it was a piece of cheesecake or something. Yes, it was cheesecake. The kind with chocolate chips and caramel and chopped pecans, and my mouth was watering just knowing I was in the same room with it. It had been years since I'd tasted cheesecake.

She had just taken a small bite and now held up one finger, chewing before she spoke. The look on her face was one of pure pleasure. Finally, she swallowed and then smiled and said, "In all things, moderation."

"What?" I asked.

While I would have eaten the whole thing in two bites, she displayed much more self-restraint. Much more grace and dignity. More...elegance. She licked her lips and then wiped the corner of her mouth with a nearby napkin. "In all things, moderation," she repeated softly.

"That sounds familiar," I said. "Where have I heard it before? Is it from the Bible or something?" It sounded Biblical, anyway. Although, I wasn't familiar enough with scripture to recognize a direct quote when I heard one, it had that Biblical ring to it.

"I don't know," she said thoughtfully. She took a sip of steaming coffee from an oversized mug and leaned back in her chair. "I've heard it somewhere, too, though."

I sat down in a chair across from her desk, thinking I could just do a Web search later if I really wanted to know.

"Or maybe it goes, 'Moderation in all things,'" she said. "I'm not sure which."

We were both CPAs at one of the larger accounting firms in the Atlanta area and though technically not "friends," we had known each other through work for some time. I had come into her office now to borrow her scissors for a science project I was working on for my son, Justin. I knew I had to be getting back to my office soon, but considering I'd tried every fad diet on the planet, I had to find out more.

Her name was Amanda Spencer and we were about the same age, early forties, but she looked much younger—a beautiful woman with smooth, flawless skin and perfect, white teeth. She always seemed cheerful and her smile was infectious whenever I ran into her in the hallways or the break room.

"But you eat all the time," I said. "It seems like every time I see you, you have a fork in your hand. It's not fair. You eat everything you want and you never seem to gain an ounce." I knew I sounded like a whiney baby, but it really didn't seem fair. All my adult life I had struggled with my weight.

"I do eat anything I want," she said. From anyone else it would have sounded smug, but from her, just sort of matter-of-fact. "And it does seem as though I'm eating all the time, but if you think about it, I really don't eat a lot."

"I don't understand," I said, folding my arms.

She gestured toward her plate. "I've been nibbling on this piece of cheesecake all morning. Someone brought in a couple of boxes and left them in the break room for everyone. There's probably some left if you want a piece."

"You've been eating that same cheesecake all morning?" I asked. "Seriously?"

"Well, that may be a slight exaggeration," she said, "but, let's see…I got in this morning at about eight-thirty." She looked down at her watch. "It's nine-forty-five now, and as you can see, there's still quite a bit left."

She was right—there was almost half of it left. I wanted to grab it and make a run for the door. But she had said there was more in the break room, hadn't she? If only I had enough willpower to keep walking past that door on my way back to my office.

"But why do you ask?" she said. "You're not overweight."

"I'm flattered," I said, waving her off. "But I know better. I could stand to lose thirty or forty pounds."

"No. Surely not," she said sincerely. "You must hide it well, then."

"Well if you notice, you rarely see me in anything but a dress or skirt and I'm usually never without a suit jacket of some sort. Even in summer."

She hugged herself and gave a faux shiver for emphasis. "Well, they keep it cold enough in here for one. I usually keep a blanket across my lap."

It was true. Even with a jacket, I never seemed to get warm enough at work. It was a common complaint within the building. Most people sat in their offices or cubicles, year-round, with portable electric heaters.

"I hear your daughter's getting married," she said.

I hated to stray so far from the subject. Did she not want to share her secret for staying so thin? Was she like those women who refuse to share their best recipes? "That's right," I answered anyway. "Only six more months."

"Really? That's great. Her name is Jennifer, right? How old is she now?"

"She's twenty-one," I said, nodding. Jennifer was from my first marriage and a good bit older than my other two children. "She graduates from college in May, so the wedding will be in September. I haven't picked out the proverbial 'mother's dress' yet. And it's an evening wedding—very formal and elegant. I really would love to lose some weight before then."

I hadn't consciously steered us back toward the subject, but I was thrilled when she said, "Well, maybe I can help you with that."

"Oh, that would be wonderful," I said. "You really wouldn't mind?"

"No, no, not at all. I'd be happy to do anything I can."

Apparently she wasn't one of "those" women. I wanted to jump up and down, but I didn't want to seem too eager. Unfortunately, it was about that time I heard the corporate receptionist calling me on the overhead pager, "Michelle Carter, please dial extension 4942. Michelle Carter, 4942."

Amanda looked at me. "That's Mr. Russell's extension, isn't it?"

I nodded. He was the CFO and our direct superior. "He's looking for that P&L statement," I said, sitting up in my chair.

She gestured toward the phone on her desk. "Do you want to use my extension?"

"Oh, no, thanks, I'll just walk down to his office." I hated to leave, though. "So, can we get together sometime and talk some more?"

"Sure," she said. "Anytime."

I felt my cell phone vibrate in my jacket pocket and knew it was Mr. Russell trying to reach me by a different route. I tried to press the mute button before the vibration changed into a full-fledged ring, but just then the phone peeled out a loud rap tune. My prankster adolescent boys were always changing my ring-tone and cranking up the volume.

I stood to leave, finally managing to silence the ringer. "Thank you," I said. "I'd really appreciate anything you could tell me." I regretted never having taken the time to get to know her before. "I'll be getting back with you, then."

On my way back to my office to pick up the P&L statement, I stopped by the break room. There was no turtle cheesecake left, but there was still almost a full box of plain old "New York." Not my favorite, but I grabbed a plastic fork and quickly shoveled two pieces onto a paper plate. I practically swallowed them whole as I sprinted down the hallway, licking my fork clean before I made it to the door.

CHAPTER 2

Circumstances with work and wedding plans kept me from speaking with her again until some three weeks later. Plus, she had been on assignment at our Dallas office for the past week. I happened to catch her in the break room early one morning.

Our break room was quite large, with a long row of cabinets to the left of the door and a large coffee maker with three carafes. It was no Starbucks, but as office break rooms go, it wasn't half-bad, and there always seemed to be a fresh pot. There were several vending machines to the right with absolutely nothing healthy in any of them.

When I walked in, her back was to me and she was casually leaning against the bottom row of cabinets, her hip propped against the edge of the countertop. She was talking softly to one of our new controllers—a nice-looking man with salt-and-pepper hair that was more salt than pepper at the temples. He had only been working with us a little over a month, but it had been said she was already involved with him. But that, of course, was none of my business. It was probably just a rumor, and they were both divorced, so it was really no one else's business either.

She looked great, as always, dressed in a simple light-colored linen shirt and darker slacks with a matching pair of casual flats. She was still nodding at something the man was saying when she turned and noticed me and smiled. "Michelle, hi, good morning."

I nodded, not wanting to interrupt.

Her companion looked at me and said, "Morning," with a tip of his head. It was only when she introduced us that I realized he had a British accent. "It's very nice to meet you," he told me. Then he politely excused himself and told her he would talk to her soon.

"How've you been?" she asked me as he walked away.

I shrugged. "Oh, I've been fine, I guess. How 'bout you?"

"I've been well." She watched the man exit through the now-closing door and raised her brows. "Very well."

But then again, I'd always believed most rumors had at least some basis in fact. "I'll bet," I said, laughing. More power to her, I thought. They made a great-looking couple.

She leaned back against the countertop, the heels of her palms resting against the slick, ivory Formica surface as she faced me. "How's the wedding coming along?" she asked.

"Not so good, actually," I said. "I'm afraid the bride-to-be may be getting cold feet."

"Uh oh," she said. "You're right, that doesn't sound good."

7

"No, it doesn't. She's given him the old 'I need space' cliché." I felt my hands involuntarily squeeze into fists. "I could just kill her."

"Oooh. That really doesn't sound good." She took her purse and cup from the countertop. Her coffee smelled of hazelnut, my favorite—but I had long ago sworn off flavored creamers. "Why don't you pour yourself a cup? Do you have time to chat?"

"Sure," I said. I really didn't, but I didn't want to pass up this chance. I quickly grabbed an insulated paper cup and filled it with decaf.

She had chosen a round table in a quiet corner of the room. "So, do you think she's just not ready to get married yet, or what?" she asked as I sat down across from her, a packet of fake creamer and a swizzle stick in hand.

"I don't know," I said, stirring the creamer into my cup. "I asked her that when he first proposed, and she convinced me she was, assuring me she was all grown up now, you know, mature for her age. And I have always believed she was. Of course, now I'm not so sure."

"Do you think maybe he's just not the one, then?"

"No, I really do believe he is. Actually, I think they're made for each other." And I was only being half facetious when I said, "He's the only one who would put up with her. She's mature, but she can be a little head-strong. They've been seeing each other for almost four years. And well, actually she hated him in the beginning. He lived in our neighborhood then, and he used to fly up and down our street in his souped-up sports car. And she would be watching the kids pass the football to each other on the front lawn or something, and she would get so furious because he was always speeding. She even nicknamed our street 'Racetrack Road' because of him."

She laughed.

"Finally, one day she hopped into her Jeep and headed out after him. She caught up to him at a stop light and somehow convinced him to pull over. They both got out of their cars and she started yelling at him, calling him every name in the book, and I think, by then, he had a few choice words for her, too. Anyway, one thing led to another, and she ended up slapping him across the face. And would you believe, before they parted ways, he had asked her out?"

"Oh, no, you're kidding. That's a riot."

"And since then, they've been head over heels in love. I'm not sure what's gotten into her now."

"So, she told him she needed space and just broke it off?"

"Pretty much, yeah," I said, taking my first sip of the still-searing-hot coffee. "We had just picked out the bridesmaid dresses. And they were so beautiful. I think I told you it was supposed to be an evening wedding?"

She nodded. "This fall, right?"

"Yes, in September. So we went with a dark blue." I described the cut of the dresses.

"Oh, they do sound pretty. How's the boy taking it? What's his name?"

"Jeremy. He's terribly upset, bless his heart." I hated that lynchpin of the southern vernacular, but I could never seem to stop myself from using it. "He's such a cute, sweet kid. He even called me, asking me to talk to her. He was crying when we hung up the phone."

"Awe, poor guy," she said sincerely. "Do you think she'll eventually come around?"

"I think she probably will. I'm hoping so, at least. At first I was against her getting married because they're both so young. You know, when we were that age, it didn't seem so young. Practically half my high-school graduating class was married or pregnant or both, by the time they graduated." I was exaggerating, of course. "And I know she loves him dearly. I can't imagine what's wrong with her. But I'm staying out of it—not advising her either way. The last thing I want to do is push her into something she isn't sure about. In the meantime, though, I've somehow managed to put on another five pounds."

Her jaw dropped. "Oh, no," she said, and she seemed genuinely concerned. "What happened?"

"Well, I thought I'd go ahead and try what you'd told me so far about your secret for staying so thin. Remember, you said you eat everything you want. Well, evidently I 'want' to eat a lot more than you do. And with the stress of the wedding and all…"

"Oh, you have had a bad few weeks then, haven't you?" She touched my forearm softly. "I'm sorry," she said. "But you have to be careful not to confuse 'anything' with 'everything.'"

"I'm sure there's a subtle difference there," I said, laughing.

"Yes, it may be subtle, but it's a very important difference. And I'll try to help you as much as I can, but I can only speak for myself—only tell you what works for me."

"I understand," I said, nodding. "That's no problem. Whatever you're doing, I can see it works well."

"You have to remember the most important thing, then."

"Okay, what is the most important thing?" I asked.

"In all things, moderation," she said. "You can't eat 'everything' you want but you can, and you should, eat 'anything' you want."

"This seems a little more complicated than I originally thought," I said.

"It's not complicated," she said. "Not at all, as a matter of fact, but there are a few guidelines you'll need to follow."

"Okay, that's no problem. Like what?" I asked.

"Well, I've been thinking since we talked last. There have been a lot of people over the years who've asked me the same thing you did, 'How do you stay so thin?' They would see me eating all the time and assume I was eating a lot, just the way you did. So, when you asked, I decided to really think it through—to make a list of everything I normally do—if you're interested."

Interested? Couldn't she see I was foaming at the mouth? "Oh, I'm definitely interested," I said. "That's great! Fantastic."

She fumbled through her purse. "It's all here on my iPhone if you want to go over it right quick."

"Yes, yes, absolutely."

"Well, I've never really consciously followed any sort of plan," she said, looking at the screen, "but I came up with about five steps I seem to follow without really thinking about it."

"Great! Five steps? I can do that. At least, I think I can."

"I'm sure you can," she said, "but if you have any health problems or anything like that, this might not be

11

such a good idea. Even though technically this isn't a quote diet, you know, all diets seem to advise you to talk to your doctor first. If you have diabetes or heart problems or anything…"

"Oh, no, nothing like that. Actually, I just had my annual physical and everything checked out fine." Our insurance plan had a wellness benefit and I rarely failed to have my yearly exam. I looked at it as money thrown away if I ever missed one—almost like giving the insurance company part of my salary and getting nothing in return.

After making a few taps on her iPhone, she said, "Okay, first of all, when I eat, I make sure it's something I really like and something I really want at the time."

"Oh, I see, by 'anything' you want, you mean you only eat what you like?"

She nodded. "And only something I want at the time."

"I get it, now. You don't eat something just because it's there. Or just because it doesn't have many calories. It has to be something that tastes good—something you really want."

"Exactly," she said, sipping her coffee. "Something I'm craving or really in the mood for. And I only eat small amounts at one time."

"That's where the 'moderation' comes in?"

"That's right," she said, nodding. "You have to eat small amounts at one time. I would say 'portions,' but that sounds too regimented. I really don't follow a regimented plan. I just sort of follow these steps subconsciously."

I spied a pen on a nearby table and hopped up to grab it. "I need to write this down," I said. Then, returning to my seat, I took a napkin from the center of the table. I hated to stay away from my desk for so long, but I eased the guilt by telling myself I'd worked so much unpaid overtime throughout the years that the company owed me a lot more time than I owed it.

She looked down at my improvised notepad. "I can just email it to you if it would be easier."

I pondered that for about a millionth of a second. No, I wanted to get it all down now. The sooner the better. After all, we could come under nuclear attack before she hit the send button. Plus, I was pretty sure I would need some elaboration. I wanted to know now whether this was something I could actually do, or if it would be like every other diet I had tried in the past where I would starve myself to lose weight, only to gain it all back again later. "Would you mind just going over it now?" I asked.

She took a sip from her cup and said, "No, that's fine. Whichever you prefer." She scooted her chair back. "Just give me a second to warm my coffee. I like it steaming hot. Can I get you some more?"

"No, mine's fine, thanks." She had only taken a few sips of hers, but I noticed her pour it out and start all over.

Across the top of the napkin, I wrote, "In All Things, Moderation," as I waited. Then I stroked the number "1" on the napkin in the blue ink and circled it.

When she sat back down, I said, "Okay, step number one is 'Eat what you want,' correct?"

"That's right," she said, nodding. "Eat what you want and only what you want."

"And only what you want," I said as I wrote each word. "Okay, and why is that so important?"

"Because you don't want to waste calories on something you don't really like or really want."

"That makes sense," I said, looking up at her.

"But make no mistake," she said, "you have to take in fewer calories than you're taking in now to lose weight, but my feeling is, why not do it with less food and more flavor?"

I considered that for a moment. I had always done things the other way around—eaten tasteless diet food and eaten lots of it. I had never thought of it like this before. "So, you eat for the taste instead of that full feeling?"

"That's right," she said. "Which is not to say you will still be hungry, you just can't allow yourself to get to that overly-full stage."

"I see," I said, nodding. Then another thought occurred to me. "But what if I only like, say, Reese's Peanut Butter Cups? That can't be very healthy."

She laughed and said, "No, I'm sure it's not. You know, you have to be reasonable. You don't want to cause yourself health problems, and you don't want your muscles to turn to mush from lack of protein or your thighs to turn to cottage cheese from too much sugar or too much fat."

I hated to tell her, but my thighs had already turned to cottage cheese some time ago.

"You can't gorge yourself on any one thing," she continued. "Remember, 'In all things, moderation.' The point is to not deny yourself any particular food. And hopefully, once you get used to eating all those foods you've denied yourself for so long, you'll find you don't crave them quite as much, and you'll start to crave healthier foods."

"I understand."

"I ate part of that cheesecake that day in my office," she continued, "but I never did finish the rest of it. And later I had some really good vegetables from downstairs and, you know, regular healthy stuff. And so far this morning I've had a banana and some walnuts and raisons."

"But you would rather have had another piece of cheesecake, though, right?"

"Well, some days I might not eat any particularly healthy foods, but some days that might be all I eat. And some days it's a mix of both. Believe it or not, I was actually craving a banana on my way in this morning, so I stopped by the little fruit-stand thingy across the street."

There was a cute little shop on the corner of two of our main downtown streets that sold not only fruit, but different kinds of nuts and other healthy treats. They also sold the most delicious brownies I had ever put in my mouth.

"Of course, I also had to get one of those fabulous brownies," she said, reading my mind. "The ones with the chocolate frosting. I'm sure you know the ones."

"Oh, I definitely know the ones."

"I haven't started on it yet, though. One thing you don't want to do is, if you decide you want to eat something healthy, eat it and then turn around and immediately eat something sweet. I've done that before. I'll be craving something healthy and then think, 'Oh, since I ate something healthy, I can eat some chocolate now.' I have to tell myself to wait until later."

"I understand," I said as I jotted it down along the margin of the napkin. "Then you end up eating too much at one time."

She nodded. "And I'll elaborate on that later under another step."

"Okay," I said. I didn't want to jump the gun. I returned to my list. "Okay, number one was 'Eat what you want and only what you want.'" Under the number one, I wrote a "2" and circled it. "And what would you consider to be number two?"

"Well normally when I eat, I only take small bites and then I chew them very slowly. And I make sure I've completely chewed and swallowed each bite before I take another."

I can do that, I thought to myself. I never had, though. As a matter of fact, there had been times I had been so hungry I'd taken two or three bites out of my hamburger before I'd even started chewing. My mouth would be so full I could hardly chew at all.

"So," she continued without looking back down at her iPhone, "number two would be 'Take small bites and chew them slowly.'"

"Take small bites and chew them slowly," I said as I wrote. I looked up at her from the napkin. I needed specifics. "Like how small?"

"Very small," she said. "It depends on what you're eating, of course, but as a general rule, I'd say no larger than a dime or nickel. And then you have to chew those bites very slowly. Do you ever watch other people eat?" she asked.

"No, I'm usually too busy shoveling food into my own mouth to pay attention to anyone else." It was my attempt at self-deprecating humor and she laughed.

"Start watching them," she said, still smiling. "Most thin people, people who stay thin at least, seem to pick at their food, push it around on their plate. It seems to grow and never seems to go away."

"People whose weight doesn't fluctuate too much, you mean?"

"Yes," she said, "people who aren't obsessed with food. And then, if you pay attention to, let's say, 'less than thin' people, they usually scarf down their food without even tasting it."

"I have to say, I'm probably one of the latter," I confessed. "But I know what you mean. We tease my husband's brother about having to count his fingers before he starts eating to make sure he still has them all when he's finished. He always eats a lot and he always eats it fast."

She laughed. "It's the same with my dog," she said, and then her eyes grew large when she realized how it sounded. "Not to compare your brother-in-law with my dog or anything. No offence…"

"No, no, none taken. What kind of dog do you have?"

"She's a Jack Russell 'terror.'"

It was clear she had used the word "terror" instead of "terrier" intentionally, and I smiled. "I've heard they can be a real handful."

"Yes, that's putting it mildly. No, I love her to death, and I know I shouldn't feed her 'people food,' but my kids started it a long time ago, and now she'll barely touch her dog food because she's always waiting for something better."

"Oh, my schnauzer is the same way," I said.

"Schnauzers are great," she said. "Much more sedate."

"But she gets doggie treats instead of people food."

"Good," she said. "Be glad you never started that. Anyway, her name is Annie, and she waits and waits for some really good people food from us, but when she gets it, she practically swallows it whole. And I can't understand why she doesn't just eat her plain old dry, bland dog food if she's not even going to take the time to taste the good stuff."

"I've never thought about it like that. You're right, Rigel eats his treats so fast, there's no way he has time to actually taste them."

"Aren't they funny," she said. "So, you want to eat something you really like—something that really tastes good—and then take the time to chew it slowly enough to really enjoy it because you don't want to waste calories on something that's going to go down so fast you don't even have time to taste it. Which leads me to number three on the list...I make sure I taste every bite, every single crumb, every morsel. I 'savor the flavor,' if you will."

"Savor the flavor," I repeated the words, and they seemed to roll off my tongue. That one would be easy to remember.

"Oh my God," she said. "I didn't realize how corny that sounded until you just said it."

"No, no, I like it," I said. "Savor the flavor." I wrote it down as number three.

"Anyway," she said, "I just make myself take the time to actually taste what I'm eating." She sipped her coffee and then looked down at her watch. "Oh, no, I didn't know it was getting so late. I have a meeting in just a few minutes and then I have a flight to Charlotte for some preliminaries on the new office up there."

"Oh, no," I said, too, "just when we were getting somewhere." That whole email thing was beginning to sound like the option I should have gone for.

"I know, I'm sorry. We'll have to get together when we have more time. Away from work."

"That would be great."

"We'll have to do lunch," she said. "I think I need to elaborate on everything before you get started. I wouldn't want you to gain any more weight because of something I haven't explained fully."

"No, no," I said, "I certainly can't afford to do that."

"I should be back in town by the end of next week. How does that look for you?"

That seemed so far away, but I was grateful for anything she was willing to share with me. Even if it had to be on her schedule. "Anytime is good for me," I said. Whatever plans I had, I knew I could change for this.

"Maybe we could meet on Saturday, then," she said. "That way we wouldn't have to worry with getting back to work."

"Saturday would be great," I said. Should I ask her to email me the rest of the list or would that sound too eager? I didn't want her to think I was just using her.

"Okay. There are only two more if you want to go ahead and write them down."

Great, I thought. Problem solved. "Yes, if you think you have time."

"I think so," she said, checking her watch again. "Okay, well another thing I do is, I stop eating when I first start to feel full. I try to never let myself get 'too' full—to never eat a lot at one time."

"So, that would be step number four, then?" I asked. "Never let yourself get too full?"

She nodded. "And by full I don't mean stuffed, you understand."

"Yes, I think so," I said. "Like we discussed earlier—you eat for the taste and not for that full feeling." I really needed some elaboration, but I knew she was in a hurry and I didn't want to push it.

"Right, I stop when I first start to feel full. And going back to number two, the slower you eat, ironically, the faster it seems to catch up with you, so the faster you'll start to feel full."

"I see. I've actually noticed that before." I hadn't actually noticed that before because I rarely ate slowly enough for that full feeling to catch up with me while I was still eating. But I had noticed the opposite. The faster I ate, the more I could hold. And usually by the time I stopped, I'd be so miserable I couldn't walk. "But what if I'm starving?" I asked. "I know me, I can't just eat a few bites and quit."

"Well, remember when you told me I seem to eat all the time but never gain weight?"

"Mm-hm," I said, nodding. "This is the first time I remember seeing you when you weren't eating."

"You're probably right," she said, laughing. "Well, not only do I not allow myself to get to the point where I'm too full, I also don't allow myself to get to the point where I'm too hungry either."

"So, that would be number five, then?"

"Yes," she said, "never let yourself get too hungry."

I wrote down the last two steps—number four, "Never let yourself get too full," and number five, "Never let yourself get too hungry." Boy, this sounded too good to be true, I thought. I could eat "all the time," just like she did, and still lose weight?

"So, you have these five steps…" I looked down at my make-shift note pad. "Eat what you want and only what you want, take small bites and chew them slowly, savor the flavor, never let yourself get too hungry, and never let yourself get too full—and they all center around this one theme, 'Moderation in all things'?"

"Yes," she said thoughtfully. "I've never thought about it quite like that, but yes, these steps enable you to achieve the 'moderation.'"

"This sounds wonderful," I said. "But there has to be a catch. I mean, you probably exercise your rear-end off, right?"

She smiled. "No, not much at all. I actually wish I could make myself exercise more. But really, the most I do is walk. I usually walk every afternoon. And I take the stairs whenever I can—things like that. I try to find some excuse to keep moving when I get home from work. I pick up around the house, cook, work in my flower bed, you know, whatever I can think of. I've always found it difficult to exercise if I'm not accomplishing something else at the same time. Like, sometimes I'll walk to the convenience store down the street from my house to grab some milk or something—whatever I'm out of—so that I'm accomplishing something else while I'm quote exercising."

I had never thought of that. Maybe that would help me, too.

"Then sometimes, if the weather's not too bad," she said, "I'll park in the lot down the street so I'll have farther to walk to the office. But as with taking the stairs, I wouldn't do it if it wasn't safe."

"Oh, no, neither would I." Our building was heavily secured as was the surrounding area. Plus, there were tons of people walking to their offices, as well.

"But I don't belong to a gym or anything like that. I find it hard to pay for exercise when there's so much of it you can get for free. Like people who join a gym and then pay someone else to do their lawns."

Uh oh, I thought. I, too, was guilty of that. Of course, I never actually went to the gym unless it was right after New Years Day. Not only was I paying for exercise I wasn't getting, I was paying the kid down the street to get his exercise, too. Not to mention the fact that I had two perfectly healthy teenagers at home who could mow the lawn instead of playing video games all the time.

"Or paying someone to do their housework," she continued. "They could kill two birds with one stone if they did their own yard work and housework, and they'd come out better financially as well. But no, I definitely recommend regular exercise. I just wish I could take my own advice on that. And believe me, I've tried. Like everybody else, I've joined a gym and been gung-ho to begin with, but it never lasted. So, I just do what I can on my own now."

"No, no, I understand."

She stood to leave. "Well, I've got to run now." She poured what remained of her coffee down the drain and dropped the cup in the nearby garbage can. "I'll see you in a couple of weeks, then. I'll call you."

"Okay," I said, walking her to the door as though she were leaving my house instead of the company break room, "that sounds great. I hope you have a safe trip, and you don't know how much I appreciate this, Amanda."

"Oh, it's no problem at all, Michelle. I'm happy to do it. Actually, it's kind of fun. It'll be interesting to see what kind of progress you make."

CHAPTER 3

I didn't do this often. Because it was so expensive, the only time I came here was for special occasions. Sometimes for birthdays or anniversaries, my daughter's high-school graduation. As a matter of fact, that was the last time I had come here, and that had been almost four years ago. But I loved this restaurant. It was a local favorite in the Buckhead area, closer to work, actually, than to where I lived. An area known for its vast, eclectic offering of food and entertainment. It was Amanda's suggestion anyway, so who was I to refuse? And wasn't this a special occasion? Hopefully, I would have something to celebrate soon.

I had never been here for lunch, though. In fact, I didn't even know they were open for lunch. I stepped under the dark green canvas awning and waited for the couple ahead of me to make it through the entrance. The man held the door open for his companion, and then waited for me to enter, as well. "Thank you," I said, allowing him to join her ahead of me. He gave the maître d' his name and then followed him to their table.

I studied the photos on the walls as I waited—photos of the owner with various well-known Americans who had obviously dined here over the years. Jimmy Carter, of course—this was Atlanta, after all. Barak Obama, George Bush, the elder, Ronald Reagan, Hillary Clinton, Morgan Freeman, Brett Favre, Oprah Winfrey, the list went on and on.

The place had been here for more than twenty-five years. I knew that because I had dated a guy in high school who was part of the wait staff. He always brought me here because we got to eat for free. And that was fine by me because the food was great even back then, and I would never have gotten to eat here otherwise because of the price. That was the first time I'd ever tasted caviar. They had a thin slice of smoked salmon on some sort of small, toasted specialty bread with cream cheese and a dollop of caviar on top. It was fantastic, and we both ordered that same appetizer every time we went out. Years later, I heard he had moved to Boston and opened his own restaurant. I hoped he was doing well.

I was about to give my name, but then I remembered Amanda had made the reservation and it would probably be in hers instead. I wasn't used to having reservations for lunch. Most of the restaurants I frequented at noon were on work days and were first come first serve—and hope the service was fast enough to get you back to the office before you had gone too far past the hour allotment.

Following the maître d' to our table now, I noticed the other diners, most dressed casually because it was a Saturday—some even in blue jeans—and since this was such a warm, early-spring day, what few children there were, all seemed to be in shorts. I had chosen slacks and a light-weight jacket. How I longed for the days when I had been able to wear blue jeans anywhere I wanted—and look damned good in them to boot. But that was many moons and many children ago. What was it about blue jeans that made you need to have a great body to look even remotely good in them? Not only did I no longer wear blue jeans, I didn't even like to wear dress pants anymore because, although they didn't do as much damage as jeans, I could definitely hide better under a dress or skirt.

The maître d' led me to a small booth large enough for only two. It was a very quiet and intimate area and I was glad. It would be much more conducive to our "intimate" diet conversation. I unfolded my napkin now and draped it across my lap. There were still a few minutes before our planned meeting time.

Our waiter was a very confident, yet friendly, young man who appeared to be in his mid-twenties. "Good afternoon," he said, looking down at his watch. "Yes, it is afternoon. Hasn't been 'after' noon for long, but afternoon, nonetheless. My name is Tom. You're waiting for someone?"

"Yes."

He handed me a menu. "Could I bring you something to drink while you wait?"

"That would be nice," I said. He was probably thinking of something alcoholic, but it was far too early for that for me, even on my day off. "I think I'll just have some iced tea, please."

"I'll bring that right out," he said, "and I'll wait until your lunch companion arrives to go over our specials."

"Very good," I said.

I had taken the seat facing the doorway so I could see her come in, but my attention was diverted to the table across the aisle from me by the delightful aroma of what appeared to be a succulent medium-well fillet. I watched as a man carefully carved out a large slice and place it into his eagerly awaiting mouth. My stomach churned. I was starving. I hadn't eaten anything all morning in anticipation of this rare treat. In fact, I hadn't even eaten so much as one bite since lunch the day before and I was wishing Amanda would hurry up and get here. Maybe I should order an appetizer, I thought.

I looked over the menu. It hadn't changed much since the last time I was here, and I had already kind of decided on the grilled tuna when Amanda had suggested the place over the phone the day before. I had been assured it was dolphin-safe the last time I had ordered it, and although I knew it was very good, in truth, I would have loved to allow myself to try something more adventurous, something tastier, with more calories. I couldn't decide if I was glad or sad to see they still hadn't removed the smoked salmon canapés from the menu. That had to be very high in calories. I hadn't had the nerve to order it since way back when.

The waiter brought my drink and as I loaded it with Splenda, I caught a glimpse of Amanda's blond hair reflecting the sunlight from the large plate-glass windows at the front of the dining room.

I was surprised by her attire. She wore a simple, white V-neck tee shirt tucked into shapely blue jeans with a brown leather belt and some kind of cute Birkenstock sandals. On most anyone else the clothes would have looked unkempt, but on her, they looked tasteful…elegant.

Amanda spoke to the maître d' and soon she was following him to our booth. I had always thought of her as pretty. She had a way of making you feel as though you were the only other person in the room, but watching her walk toward me now, it was surreal. And the men, oh my God, they literally stopped mid-conversation, mid-bite and watched as she walked by. She had gotten a touch of sun and her skin positively glowed, and I was fairly certain no one would ever believe she was forty-something years old.

"I'm sorry I didn't dress any better," she said, sitting down across from me. "Gavin had back-to-back soccer games this morning."

"Oh, no, you look great. As always," I added. "If I looked that good in blue jeans, that's all I would wear."

"Oh, I'm sure you look fine," she lied.

"Well no, but hopefully after this, I'll be able to pass the blue jean test," I said. "Gavin's your youngest, right?"

"Yes, he's sixteen. You have one about that age, too, don't you?"

I nodded. "William just had his fifteenth birthday Sunday. Then there's Justin who's thirteen."

"And you said Jennifer was twenty," she paused, trying to remember, "twenty-two?"

"Almost," I said. "She'll be twenty-two next month." Although she didn't say anything, I knew she must be wondering about the age gap between my daughter and my two sons. "She's from a previous marriage," I volunteered. "One of those 'shotgun weddings' that usually don't work out."

She nodded, smiling. "I had a couple of close calls with that, myself."

The waiter appeared out of nowhere. "Mrs. Spencer," he said surprised, looking down at Amanda.

"Tom," she said. "How are you?" Evidently she frequented the place much more often than I did.

"I-I'm good," he sputtered. The confident air he had displayed earlier seemed to have disappeared. "How are you? Can I get you something to drink?" He fumbled with the menu, and then managed to place it before her. Clearly this young man was infatuated with her.

"I'm doing great," she said. "Yes, I think I'll have a Sprite."

Not a Diet Sprite, not a Sprite Zero, not a Fresca—although I wasn't sure they even made those anymore—just a plain old high-fructose corn syrup, Sprite.

"I'll get that right out to you." He looked at me. "And I'll get you a refill on your tea," he said.

"Thank you," I replied.

"So, is the wedding back on?" she asked as he walked away.

"No," I said regretfully. "Things have gotten worse, actually."

She leaned in toward me, clasping her hands together on the table. "Oh, no, what's happened?"

"Well, you know I told you she had broken things off because she needed her so called 'space?' And how he was devastated and calling me and crying and everything?"

"Mm-hm," she said, nodding.

"Well, you're not going to believe this…"

"Oh, no, what?"

"He's started dating someone else."

"You're kidding. Wow! That was awfully fast."

"I know! I think he's probably just doing it to bring her to her senses. You know, to try to make her wake up and smell the coffee."

"I'm sure you're right," she said. "I don't think you can turn it on and off that quickly. If he actually really cared for her."

"Well, that's just it," I said. "Now she's fully convinced he never cared for her at all. I don't believe that. I believe he was sincere but, you know, you can only take so much. Now the shoe is on the proverbial other foot. She's the one who's crying now."

Tom returned and set our drinks before us. He had not displayed much evidence of a southern accent earlier, and absolutely no trace of one now as he went over the specials, his confidence fully regained. "Today, we have a superb loup de mer in a divine squid sauce. Also, a delectable foie gras with chanterelles and balsamic vinegar. And we also have a pearl pasta risotto with fresh asparagus and butternut squash. But I suggest a new dish our chef is trying out today—pan seared sea scallops over sautéed couscous with a delicate, white, garlic-butter sauce. It's absolutely fabulous."

"It sounds fabulous, Tom," Amanda said, handing him her menu. "In fact, I think that's what I'll have."

"And do you want your usual blue cheese dressing?" he asked.

"Yes, please."

He looked at me. "I'll have the grilled Tuna," I said dully, looking down at the menu. "What kind of low-calorie dressing do you have?"

"We have a light raspberry vinaigrette that's very good."

"That will be fine," I said.

He nodded. Like any good waiter, he had no need to write anything down. "And would either of you like to start out with an appetizer?" he asked. He looked at Amanda. "We have your favorite—soft shell crab nuggets with Hollandaise."

"Oh, no thank you," she said. "Not today."

Then, looking at me, he said, "How about you, ma'am?"

"I believe I would like something," I said without thinking. As hungry as I was, I couldn't possibly wait for the entrée. "I'd like the smoked salmon with caviar."

"Excellent choice," he said, taking our menus, "excellent choice. I'll be back with that shortly."

When he was gone, Amanda started back where we'd left off, "So, Jennifer's pretty upset, then?"

I nodded. "And even though I know she probably brought it on herself," I said, "it breaks my heart to see her like this. She can't eat or sleep. She gets the fork halfway to her mouth and has to put it back down. Now that's a diet plan."

"Oh, I know exactly what you mean," she said. "I was so miserable during my divorce that all I could eat was chicken soup. And I had trouble even keeping that down. I hate to see anybody go through that."

"I do, too. She's up all night on the phone with her friends, crying. She won't leave the house. It's just awful."

"Have you spoken to…Jeremy about it?" she asked.

"No, he's stopped calling me. Feeling guilty, I guess. Or maybe he really is over her. And she forbids me to talk to him. And in the meantime, deposits have been made, hotel rooms reserved, the invitations have come in. I never cancelled them, thinking she would change her mind and then, when this happened, I forgot to call the printers. It's just a disaster. Which, none of that matters. I just want her to be happy."

"If I were you, I'd get in touch with the boy," she said. "You know, just talk to him and see what he's really thinking. Jennifer would never have to know."

"I've thought about that," I said. "And I might go ahead and do it. Just for my own peace of mind. I would hate to think he was that shallow. To be able to go from one to the other so quickly."

"No, I think it's probably like you said. He's probably just trying to bring her to her senses. Hopefully, everything will work itself out."

I nodded. I didn't know why, but I truly believed it would. "But wedding or no wedding, I still want to do this," I said. "I want to change my life. Get off the fad-diet roller coaster."

"Oh, by all means," she said. "Just trying to lose weight for a special occasion is never the way to go."

"I know," I said. "And that's what I've done all my life. I've always had some reason that I needed to lose weight very fast. In reality, I just never had enough patience to wait. I've tried liquid diets, pills, fasting, low carb, you name it. But if I had taken the time to learn how to eat the right way from the beginning, I wouldn't be having this problem now. So, instead of speeding up my weight loss, in the long run, I actually slowed it down."

"That's true," she agreed. "Those types of diets are great for quick weight-loss, but eventually you have to go back to eating normal food again, and the weight just comes back. If you follow this, though, I believe you'll still lose weight surprisingly fast—and be able to keep it off—because it's simply a new way of eating. It isn't cumbersome. You don't have to prepare a separate meal. You aren't denying yourself the foods you love. You can eat at any restaurant. I don't know—it's a suit you can wear, so to speak. Something comfortable you can live with."

I nodded. "You know, I was thinking…I've been with the company for ten years and you started not long after I did, didn't you?"

"Yes," she said. "I've been there for almost a decade. Whew, it sounds like a long time when I say it like that."

"And during that time, my weight has gone up and down thirty to forty pounds and never once stayed the same. And yours has never varied in the slightest during the whole ten years. You look just the same as the day you started."

She let out a hearty laugh. "Well, I wouldn't say that. You don't see me in the mirror getting dressed every morning."

"But your weight, it never fluctuates, does it?"

"Never more than three or four pounds," she said, "no, you're right. I actually weigh about the same as I weighed when I graduated from college." She wasn't being smug, just stating a fact.

"That's fantastic," I said. "And it's all because of this method of eating you've followed for all these years." It wasn't a question—it was the obvious answer. It wasn't a "diet," it was a way of life for her and I wanted it to be the same for me.

CHAPTER 4

Tom brought the salmon appetizer and placed it between us and then asked if he could bring us anything else. We both said we were fine.

"That looks wonderful," Amanda told me as he left.

"Oh, please, have some," I said, gathering one of the servings onto my unused fork. I shoveled it onto one of her small plates that were part of the table setting.

"All right. You talked me into it. I don't think I need a whole one, though."

"No, go ahead," I said. "I can't eat all of them, anyway." I had been hungry when I arrived but now, after inhaling the indescribable aroma from the other tables, I was absolutely ravenous. I was actually quite sure I could eat all four of them with no trouble at all, but I didn't want to seem too greedy.

I dug in, and the flavor was even better than I had remembered. But by the time I looked up, I was halfway into my last canapé which I hadn't bothered to taste after the first bite. Amanda, however, had barely touched hers. She had peeled the thin layer of crust from around the mini-toast and left it lying on the plate while she picked up the remainder with her fingers and took what looked to be only her second bite.

She was still chewing when she said, "This is great. I don't know why I've never tried it before."

I finished what was left of mine as I told her about how it had been my favorite when I'd come here in my younger days with my old boyfriend.

And when Tom brought the salads, he asked if he could take our plates. Mine of course was empty, but Amanda still had a good bit of hers left. "I think I'll keep mine," she said. "I might want to nibble on it later."

The salmon had barely put a dent in my appetite, so I inhaled the salad almost as rapidly as I had the appetizer, only taking time out to covet the sumptuous-looking clumps of blue cheese clinging to the hearts of romaine that lay on Amanda's salad plate.

She continued her nibbling as we talked about my husband Bill's heart problems, Gavin's soccer aspirations, her older son Caleb's football scholarship, and how she was indeed seeing the new office controller—all this during the time it took the waiter to bring our entrées.

As he placed them before us and took our salad plates—a good portion of hers remaining untouched—he asked if we needed anything else and we both declined.

"Thanks, Tom," she told him, surveying her meal. "This looks delicious."

"Great," he said. "I'll be back to check on you guys later. Enjoy."

The cut of albacore was about the size of a large filet—with grill marks crisscrossing its pink outer layer and under it was a hearty portion of angel-hair pasta. I couldn't wait to dig in. I chiseled off a large chunk with my knife and shoved it into my mouth as politely as I could, considering the fact that I was still famished—even after inhaling both the salmon and the salad.

I looked at her plate. The scallops were fried to a crisp honey color and they somehow managed to stay afloat in the luxurious white sauce. The couscous appeared to be tender and succulent as it dripped garlicky butter from her fork. "That looks heavenly," I said as soon as I had chewed enough to speak intelligibly.

"Oh, it's absolutely amazing," she said, nodding. "Would you like a taste?"

"No, no, this is fine," I said. "It's quite good, actually." After a few minutes of cutting and chewing, I looked down to discover that three quarters of my meal was gone. I was mortified. I glanced over at her plate and realized she had taken only a few bites. Had I not considered any of her suggestions about moderation? Well, we had agreed I wouldn't start the five steps until I had all the details, hadn't we?

After I swallowed, I stopped and watched her as she cut into one of the tender scallops with her fork. The bite was only about the size of a nickel, as she'd said it should be, and then she dipped it into the buttery sauce. She put it in her mouth and the look on her face was one of sheer ecstasy. I thought I heard a slight "ummmm" coming from her way, but that might have just been my imagination.

"Oh my God," she said. "This really is incredible."

I took my glass, and sitting back, continued chewing but more slowly, and then sipped my iced tea. "Okay," I said, "what all did I do wrong?"

"Wrong?"

"Well, I'm almost finished eating and you've barely started," I said. "I know, 'In all things, moderation,' right? I've eaten way too much already. But I have a feeling that, even if I went ahead and finished this now, I would still be craving something else."

She took another bite and then sat back in her seat, as well. After a long moment of chewing and savoring, she said, "Okay, let me ask you this...Why did you order the grilled tuna?"

"Uh, well, I was thinking it was probably the least fattening thing on the menu. And probably the healthiest thing on the menu. The least likely to make me put on more pounds. God knows I don't need any more."

"And healthy is good," she said, nodding. "Don't get me wrong. Healthy is great, if that's what you're in the mood for. There are many times when I feel like eating healthy and I would probably order the same thing. The difference is, I would order it because it was what I wanted at the time—maybe because I might be craving some balance..."

"It wasn't what I really wanted," I said. "I see where you're going."

She nodded. "Normally, I don't go for something just because it has fewer calories than anything else. Now, if it is what I'm in the mood for and it happens to have fewer calories, then by all means, that's what I order."

"I see," I said, nodding. "Rule number one, 'Eat what you want and only what you want.' But I really do like this grilled tuna."

"Oh, so do I," she said, sitting up to carve another small bite from her scallops. "I've ordered that same dish here before and been perfectly delighted."

"But still, it wasn't what I really wanted this time."

"Exactly," she said, the fork poised to enter her mouth. "If I hadn't been in the mood for the tuna and ordered it anyway, I would have left here full, but still wanting something else. Full, but empty at the same time. And then I probably would have eaten a lot of something I really wanted to make up for it. To try to satisfy that craving—to hit that spot, so to speak."

I nodded. "As soon as I heard the waiter describe the specials, I immediately wanted the scallops."

"And so did I," she said, chewing. "I'd rather eat a little of something I really want than lots of something I don't really want."

"That makes sense," I said.

Tom returned with refills on our drinks and I reloaded mine with Splenda. Amanda had barely touched hers, however, and declined. "So, you don't deny yourself anything, then?" I asked her when he'd gone. "Ever?"

She thought for a long moment. "Not really, no," she said. "If I do then, as I said, I'm never really quite satisfied. But again, remember you can't confuse 'anything' with 'everything.'"

"I understand," I said, moving the remainder of the tuna around on my plate, determined not to eat another bite. "And I know what you mean about trying to find a substitute for something you're craving, too. The other day, I remembered the kids had some leftover Reese's from Easter—yes, unfortunately they still get Easter baskets at their age. Anyway, of course I had to force myself not to dig into them. Instead, I ate about ten pounds of rice cakes trying to satisfy the craving."

"That's a lot of rice cakes," she said, laughing. "Did it work?"

"Not at all, I was still craving the candy, so I ate some diet granola bars. By that time, I was stuffed, but I still wanted the candy. Then I ended up raiding their stash just before I went to bed."

"Oh, no. And you probably felt guilty for it afterwards, too."

"All night long," I said. "I hated myself for it."

"But if you'd gone ahead and eaten a few bites of the candy, you would have consumed a lot less calories."

"Oh, no doubt," I said. "And been a lot less miserable."

"That's my problem," she said. "I have no willpower at all. Zero. And that's why I think this works so well for me. The only willpower you need is the willpower to eat in moderation, not the willpower to resist a particular food. But don't get me wrong, I'm not trying to encourage you to eat candy," she said. "I'm just saying that for me, anything in moderation doesn't seem to affect my weight."

I gestured toward her glass. "And I noticed you ordered a Sprite. Do you usually drink sodas?"

"Well not only do I eat what I want," she said, "I also drink what I want—with meals, anyway. Sometimes I might have iced tea, as you did. And I also sweeten with Splenda or whatever artificial sweetener is available."

"Really? That surprises me."

"Yes, I got used to that a long time ago. I found that real sugar is almost impossible to dissolve in a cold drink, so I started using artificial sweeteners and that's what I've kept doing."

"I've gotten used to drinking diet drinks," I said. "I don't think I could go back to regular sodas. They're too sweet. Too sugary."

"No, no, you shouldn't then," she said. "You should keep drinking diet drinks, if that's what you like. But even with those, I would still take small sips and actually take the time to taste them. I try never to over-indulge in anything, even if it is low in calories."

"Even if it's low cal?"

"Yes, everything I eat or drink, I do it in moderation. And I would advise that when you're really thirsty, to drink water. I think most people guzzle when they're really thirsty. I know I do. And it's such a waste to guzzle something that actually tastes good. I try never to drink anything but water when I'm really thirsty."

"Do you ever drink diet sodas?" I asked.

"No," she admitted, "that's one thing I've never developed a taste for. Today, I was in the mood for something light, so I ordered the Sprite. But normally if I drink a soft drink, I only take a few small sips. Then it usually gets watered down and I pour that out and start over. I don't necessarily drink one every day and I never drink very much on any given day."

"So, I should drink diet sodas in moderation? And eat low-calorie foods in moderation? Why?"

"Well for me, I just hate that overly-full feeling no matter what I eat or drink. Plus, I would think it would be hard to maintain the habit of eating in moderation if you stuff yourself when you eat low-calorie foods."

"It sounds logical," I said.

She took a small nibble from the salmon that was still on her plate and savored it for a moment. "But as I was saying, if there's a particular food I like and it happens to be a 'diet' food, then by all means, I eat it. Though, I must confess there aren't very many diet foods I really like."

I had to laugh because I felt the same way. Although the taste had definitely improved from years ago, there was just something about a food that said "diet" or "low-fat" or "low-carb" that made it seem to not taste quite as good.

"Anything goes," she continued. "Whatever I'm in the mood for. But even with low calorie foods that I happen to like, I always keep quantity in mind. I always keep 'moderation' in mind. I eat for the taste but I never eat a lot at any one time. I try to eat only the things that please me. And I never, never save the best for last."

"Oh, no," I squealed. "I always do that. Why not?"

"Well," she said, "because it's pretty much a given that you're going to eat it, even if you're full. For example, I really don't like the outside of a cinnamon roll, so I pull off the outer layers and eat only the inside. That soft sugary, buttery center. I eat it very slowly and really get into the taste of it. Then instead of eating the harder outside, I throw it away."

I gestured toward her appetizer plate. "I noticed you pulled the crust off your bread."

"Yes, it's the same for bread. I really don't like the crust, so I peel it off. I only eat the good parts of anything," she explained. "Like pizza—I mostly eat the toppings and leave the crust. Occasionally I will eat a little of the crust, but mostly just the toppings."

"Oh, I've always wanted to do that," I confessed. "But I guess I thought it seemed, I don't know, against the rules."

"Well, you kind of have to adopt that 'anything goes' approach," she said. "Break the rules."

"I think I can do that," I said. I sipped my tea. "So, you said you only eat what you want, and we both happened to love this restaurant, but what if you're with a group and they all decide to go to a restaurant you don't particularly like?"

"Well, I've actually been in that situation before," she said. "When that happens, if there's absolutely no entrée on the menu that I'm in the mood for, I will try to find an appetizer or dessert I like and have that for my meal."

"You're kidding? You eat dessert for lunch?"

"Sometimes," she said, nodding. "Sometimes for breakfast, even. Like I said, anything goes. If there's still nothing I want, I find something I can tolerate and eat just enough of it to keep myself from getting so hungry that I overeat when I finally reach something I really do like."

"So, I did right by ordering the salmon, then? I had been craving it ever since you suggested we meet here."

"Yes, then, that was good," she said. "And I can see why you were craving that. It's delicious. I try not to eat something just because it's what somebody else wants. I guess that's one of the advantages of being the 'chief cook and bottle washer' at home—I get to plan the menu. But if there's nothing I want at a particular restaurant, I just try not to go there. Most people say, 'It doesn't matter to me,' when you're trying to decide on a place to eat. When that happens, I always take the opportunity to choose a place I like."

I nodded. "That sounds like a good idea," I said. "But if I'm eating something I really love, I'm afraid I might not be able to chew it slowly enough."

"Well remember, the faster you eat it, the faster it's gone," she said. "I try to keep each bite in my mouth as long as I can for that very reason—the faster I eat it, the faster it's gone. And then I'm left with wanting more."

I knew it was going to be so hard to resist shoveling my food down, even when I wasn't starving. But she was right—I had never thought of it that way—it would just be gone faster.

"It's like we were talking about the other day," she said. "People crave something for so long and then scarf it down without even tasting it—get rid of it as fast as possible—instead of trying to make it last as long as possible. And it may take some time for you to get used to it. Even I have to remind myself from time to time."

"No kidding, really? That makes me feel better. So, it was good that I ordered the salmon, but I shouldn't have inhaled it the way I did."

"Well, probably not," she said diplomatically.

"I was just so hungry I shoveled it in."

"That's why, even if you do get to the point where you're starving, you have to concentrate on taking small bites and chewing them slowly. You want to make sure you eat slowly enough for your brain to catch up with your body. And sometimes that may take a while."

"My husband always tells me how great my meals are, and then he eats them so fast, there's no way he can even taste them. I might spend all day cooking an elaborate dinner, and then it's gone in a matter of minutes."

"Oh, my kids are the same way. They're human garbage disposals."

"I can't really say anything. I mean, look how I massacred this tuna."

"But you're about to change all that," she said.

"I hope so."

CHAPTER 5

She took another small bite of the pasta and added just a touch of a golden scallop. Then she closed her eyes and you could literally watch her face change.

"Oh my God," she said, "you've just got to taste this. It really is absolutely divine."

"Okay," I said, smiling. I'd actually been wishing she would offer again.

"I may have waited until it cooled off too much," she said. She carved out a large portion of couscous with a few healthy-looking crispy scallops and dumped it all onto a semi-clean spot on my plate.

"Oh, that's too much," I squealed.

"No, no, there's no way I'm going to eat all of this. Please, they give you entirely too much food here."

"Okay," I said. It was too late anyway—it was already on my plate. I had a feeling what little remained of my tuna was absolutely safe from me now.

I tried to do as she had done. I cut the edge off one of the scallops she had given me, and then I gathered up a small amount of the pasta onto my fork with it and put it in my mouth and slowly slid the fork out.

The combination of tastes exploded in my mouth and I knew then that she was right. The rich flavor was utterly and truly superb. The scallop was light and crisp and seared to perfection, and the garlic melded with the butter to perform an exotic tango on the surface of my tongue. I closed my eyes and concentrated on the sensation and felt as if I'd died and gone to heaven. It was still slightly warm but I had the feeling that, even cold, it would still be amazing. And for the first time in my life, I wasn't trying to hurry up and swallow so I could shove another bite into its place. I chewed this bite. I savored this bite. I fell in love with this bite. And the flavor seemed to go on forever. And it was truly a wonderful experience.

She was quiet as I explored. I went through the same motions with the next bite, somehow expecting a different result. Surely, I wouldn't be able to chew this one as slowly as the last. Surely, I wouldn't celebrate the taste as I had with the first bite. Surely, I would chew it a couple of times and swallow and it would be gone. But again, I held the bite in my mouth, swirled it around, delighted in the magnificent combination of flavors, relished each individual ingredient and then began to chew. I was already full from the tuna, but now I was also beginning to feel satisfied. Not just in my stomach. I was beginning to feel satisfied in my brain.

After the third bite, I was actually able to stop eating, actually able to leave what remained—even though it was absolutely delicious. And I found myself wishing I hadn't eaten the tuna at all, wishing I could rewind the clock and order the scallops, wishing I could start over.

I realized I had never actually taken the time to taste my food. I was always trying to finish the current bite so I could hurry and get the next one into my mouth. And now, when I thought about it, it was just as she'd said—it didn't make any sense because it would just be gone faster.

"That was unbelievable," I said, wiping my mouth. "I think I tasted the first slice of this tuna, but I don't even remember another single bite."

"Yes," she said. "It's because, not only did you eat it so fast, you probably weren't thinking about the way it tasted while you were chewing?"

"No, I wasn't concentrating on the taste at all."

"As I said before, you have to eat for the flavor, not that full, stuffed feeling. At least, that's the way I look at it. You have to ask yourself if you had rather eat lots of something you don't really want or a little of something you really love."

"I'd much rather eat the things I love."

"So had I," she said. "And I try to remember to concentrate on how good it tastes. Even if I have to say 'yummmm' to myself with every bite. I delight in the taste."

I looked down at my plate. "And instead of concentrating on the flavor of this tuna, I was thinking about everything except the taste. Thinking about my daughter and all her problems, thinking about profit and loss statements, thinking about what I'll make for dinner tonight."

"Do you remember Louise Kelly who used to work in receivables?"

"Yes," I said, wondering where she was leading, "she moved to New York or L.A. or somewhere, didn't she?"

"Mm-hm, L.A.," she said, nodding. "I used to laugh—she would be craving chocolate ice cream all day, but she'd try her best to resist it. Then she would break down and go to that little kiosk thingy downstairs and get two huge scoops. Then she would devour it while we were in a meeting or something. She would eat it so fast she'd get a brain freeze. And the whole time, she'd be talking or taking notes or going over a spreadsheet. A few minutes later she'd pick up her ice cream cup and it would all be gone. Then she would make a big frown and whine, 'Who ate my ice cream?'"

I laughed. "Oh, I do that all the time—eat something and look down and it's all gone."

"Well, one thing I find helpful is to tell myself, 'This is the last bite,'" she said. "Kind of like a smoker who's trying to quit. They have to have that last cigarette or they never have a sense of closure. If I'm eating something that's really delicious, I have to tell myself, 'This is my last bite.' And sometimes I have to say it more than once. But my point is, you have to stop when you begin to feel full."

I saw our waiter approaching through the corner of my eye. "Can I take your plate?" he asked me.

"Yes, I think so," I said, picking it up and handing it to him. I moved out of the way to let him gather up everything else. I hated to see the last scallop leave, but there wasn't enough left to take home, and I was too full to eat another bite.

He reached for Amanda's plate. "Shall I wrap this up for you?" he asked—knowing what her answer would be.

"Yes, thank you," she said, sitting back in the booth to give him room.

Standing there, holding our plates he said, "Are you ladies ready for dessert?"

I shook my head. "None for me, thank you."

He looked at Amanda. "Ms. Spencer?"

"Not yet, Tom," she said. "I would like a cup of coffee, though."

"Sure. And would you like your usual shot of Baileys on the side?"

"No, no," she said. "I think it's a bit too early for that today. Just cream will be fine."

He turned to me. "Would you like a cup, as well?"

"Yes, please," I said. "With cream, also."

"Where were we?" she asked as he walked away.

"We were talking about being able to stop eating even if something is really good."

"Well, sometimes I find comfort in telling myself I can have some more in a little while," she said. "As long as I know I can eat the rest of it later, I don't have a problem stopping when I start to feel full. And that's also incentive not to go ahead and finish it now. Just like with the scallops. I just have to tell myself, 'It's not gone. I can have some more in a little while.'"

"That will definitely be helpful."

"Or if it's something I can't eat later, I have to tell myself I can order it again next time. As with something like cheesecake, you just have to realize this is not the last cheesecake you'll ever eat, so you don't have to eat a whole piece."

"I've never thought of it like that before," I said. "I could have the rest later or some more another day."

"And that's why you have to really like what you're eating. You can't really 'savor the flavor' if you're eating something that's not exceptionally good. That's another reason it pays to eat the best parts first instead of saving them for last. That way you're full by the time you get to the not-so-good parts and you don't have to eat them."

"I can see that," I said, nodding.

"You can't allow food to be your obsession," she said, "—the only thing you think about. And if you're eating what you want, and eating it slowly and really enjoying it, it should become less and less so."

"Food is definitely my favorite obsession," I admitted.

She seemed to grow more serious. "But I can't overemphasize how important it is to savor every morsel," she said, "every…crumb. You have to find a way to think about the taste even when you're talking or doing something else."

Tom set a brushed-nickel cream pitcher down between us, and I noticed steam wafting up from the top. They even pre-heated the cream here? Apparently so. Not quite a latte, but pretty close. I didn't normally order coffee at dine-in restaurants. But this was different from my normal routine. Truly a "culinary experience," I decided.

"It's the same thing for reading," she continued. "I see people in restaurants all the time, reading. I would never be able to concentrate on both."

Tom carefully placed our steaming coffee before us and surprised me when he spoke up, "Yeah, I don't know what it is about eating alone in public," he said, then clamped his mouth shut. "Oh, I'm sorry, I didn't mean to interrupt."

"No, not at all, Tom," Amanda said. "I'll bet you see that a lot."

"I do," he said. "People just seem to feel the need to be reading if they're by themselves."

She nodded. "And actually they would be better off to just eat and luxuriate in their food."

"Yes," he agreed. "And I don't mean to boast, but the food here is just too good to be concentrating on a newspaper." He gathered our watered-down drinks and then asked if he could bring us anything else and we both declined.

I poured a dab of the warm cream into my cup. "I must admit I rarely ever think about what I'm eating after the first bite or two."

"It really takes discipline to concentrate on every bite," she said. "Especially if you're doing something else or your mind is preoccupied with other things. Sometimes if I can't concentrate, I either have to stop what I'm doing or stop eating." She poured a large splash of cream into her cup and began stirring. "I'm just trying to say that if I try to read or watch TV or anything, I can't savor the flavor. Like Louise, I look down and all my food is gone, and I want to go back and refill my plate and start over."

"Oh, I understand," I said.

"I want the flavor to have my undivided attention. And people will invariably talk to you while you're eating. I mean, it's such a social thing. You kind of have to develop a way to concentrate on the taste and the conversation—which isn't easy to do. Just like I'm yammering your ear off right now…"

"No, it's the other way around," I said. "You can't have been able to concentrate much the whole time we've been here. I'm sure it's been hard to pay attention to the flavor while you've been trying to give instructions to me."

"Oh, no, it's been fine. That's why we're really here."

CHAPTER 6

She idly watched the coffee spin as she swirled her cup. "Not only does it take full concentration to savor the flavor," she said, "it also takes concentration to recognize that full feeling. For some reason it has a lag time. And then, before you know it, you have that stuffed, miserable feeling."

"Yeah, I've always had problems with that," I admitted. "I always end up miserable after I've had a meal. But part of my problem is knowing I'm eating too much and continuing to eat anyway."

"Oh, that part is crucial," she said. "You have to stop when you first start to feel full."

"So, there's a fine line between actually being hungry and being satisfied, then?" I asked.

"Yes, there is," she said. "But if you take small bites and chew them very slowly and savor the taste, you'll begin to feel satisfied before you've eaten so much. And that's when you have to stop—when you first start to feel full."

"That could be a long time for me."

"Maybe you could practice leaving something for later. Maybe take out your normal amount then take out less and less, leaving some on your plate each time."

Wow, I thought, that did sound like a good idea. "I'll definitely have to try that."

"Of course, you can't take out more than normal just to be able to leave some."

"No, I guess that would defeat the purpose," I said. "So, about how many calories do you eat a day?"

"Well, I don't really even keep up with calories, and some days I may eat more than others. I just know that if I've followed these steps, then I haven't eaten too much. And you have to take in fewer calories than you burn to lose weight. But as I said, I'd just rather do it with less food than with less flavor."

Tom brought us each a fresh cup of coffee and more cream. I waited until he left and then finally asked her what I'd been meaning to ask her all along, "So, how did you get started in all this?"

"Well, it took a while for me to finally catch on," she said, pouring cream into her cup. "But when I was in middle school, I remember going to Wendy's…"

"You mean you've been eating like this since you were in middle school?" I asked.

"No, no," she said, taking a sip. "Like I said, it took a while for me to finally catch on. That's just about the time I first began to be conscious of my weight."

"I see," I said, nodding, stirring.

"And I was kind of chubby—you know how kids get before they hit that growth spurt?"

"Yes, they seem to have to grow wide before they can grow tall." I gingerly took a sip of scorching hot coffee. "I can't imagine you being chubby, though."

"Believe me, I was," she said. "But don't get me wrong, I'm not recommending fast food, by any means…"

"I understand," I said. "But it's not off limits."

"Well I honestly don't eat a lot of fast food anymore, so I can't really advise you on that. But I would think the same theory would apply—that it's okay in moderation, but you'll have to use your own discretion in that area."

"I usually go through the drive-through on my way home from work," I admitted. "But only when I know I don't have time to cook. Which is probably the worst time—in the evening."

"You're probably right," she said, nodding.

"But go ahead, I didn't mean to interrupt. You were at Wendy's…"

"Yes," she said, continuing, "I was at Wendy's with my softball team, and there was one girl who was with us who was thin and petite. I didn't know her all that well, I mean, we weren't close friends or anything, but she had an all-around great body. I'd seen her at a swim party the week before and was immediately envious."

"Oh, believe me, I know that feeling."

"Anyway, we had all wolfed down our burgers and fries and were ready to leave, and I looked down at her food in front of her, and she had only eaten about half of it. And I was thinking, 'Oh, no, we're going to have to sit here and wait until she finishes—we were in a tournament and had another game soon, so I was antsy."

I smiled, trying to picture her as a young girl, full of energy and rearing to go.

She continued, "But then she just got up and gathered her stuff together. And then I felt bad because we had been playing all morning and I knew she couldn't have eaten since breakfast, so I said, 'No, don't get up, finish eating.' And she said, 'That's okay, I'm finished, I'm full.' And she just got up and tossed her food in the trash."

"And the rest of you had eaten twice as much as she had in the same amount of time?"

"That's right," she said. "But she was full because she had eaten so much slower than we had."

"And she just threw the rest of it away?"

She was nodding. "I was kind of in shock because I was always taught not to throw away food, you know, 'clean your plate,' and all that."

"Yes, I was brought up the same way," I said. "And now you hear mothers tell their children, 'Make a happy plate.'"

"Or 'You can't have dessert until you finish eating everything on your plate.'"

I had always considered my upbringing to be part of my problem. "And all that does is make for fat children and obese adults," I said.

"You're so right," she said, still nodding. "Anyway, I ran into the girl again a couple of years ago, and she was still thin, still petite, and I think she had like three kids or something."

"Wow, that's great."

"And I'm not condoning throwing food away just for the sake of throwing it away," she said, "but you know, you're wasting it anyway if you eat it when you've already had enough."

"And then it ends up costing you more in health issues or costing you more to get it off your thighs at the gym."

"You're right, it does," she said, nodding. "And there are ways to keep from wasting too much. Like not taking out as much or asking for smaller servings or giving someone an extra large taste, as I did with you."

"Ha!" I laughed. I knew she had given me a lot, but I'd just thought she was being generous. "I didn't even catch on."

"And of course, asking for a to-go box."

"Yeah, I noticed Tom asked you if he could wrap yours up. I guess he didn't ask me, for obvious reasons." There was almost nothing left.

She smiled.

"But I think some people are embarrassed to ask for a doggie bag," I said. "I've never had a problem with it, it's just a rare occasion that I have enough left over to take home."

She laughed.

"But what if you're not going straight home, though?" I asked.

"Well as a rule, at least in summer, I keep a cooler in the back of my vehicle for soccer drinks anyway—Gatorade, water, sodas, and that's where I usually store my leftovers until I get home. And in winter, if it's cloudy, the car is usually cold enough to keep it cool. If not, I'll normally ask for smaller portions, or like I did with you, give whomever I'm eating with an extra-large taste. And of course, we have the refrigerator in the break room at work."

That will come in handy, I thought.

"Personally I hate to throw out food," she continued, "but I will if it's something I don't like, or if

I'm finished, and for whatever reason, I can't eat it later. At home, if I've somehow filled my plate too full, I usually cover it with Saran Wrap and shove it into the frig and then eat some of it later, and then some of it again even later."

"My kids scavenge everything so I don't think throwing away food will be a problem."

She smiled and then became thoughtful. "It seems like my kids are never home anymore. Caleb started at Wake Forest last fall, so I hardly ever see him. But sometimes I leave my leftovers in the refrigerator and they're mysteriously gone by morning. I'm pretty sure Gavin raids the frig at night when he comes in."

"Now, Bill is a different story," I said, referring to my husband. "He needs to lose weight even worse than I do, so I'll have to make sure my leftovers don't fall into the wrong hands."

She laughed and said, "Good idea."

"What about all-you-can-eat buffets?"

"They are not your friend," she said, smiling. "I try to avoid them all together, but if I do end up at one, I try to take out a very small amount of each thing I like, or think I might like, and just kind of taste everything. I eat the same way I would at any dinner table. The bad part is, you can't take anything home for later, so you can't tell yourself, 'I can have more of this when I get home.' But you can always go back another day. I'm the kind of person all-you-can-eat restaurants make money on, but that's okay. You can look around and see the huge piles of food on plates and think to yourself, 'all of those people are going to be miserable tonight,' and be glad you're not one of them."

"Not to mention the heartburn," I said, remembering the many occasions when I was one of "those people."

"That's a whole other story," she said. "Once you begin to eat less and relax and chew slowly, you should find you have less heartburn. At least that's the way it works for me. If I, for some reason, find myself overeating or eating too fast, invariably I get a touch of heartburn or indigestion—whatever you want to call it. But if I take my time and stop before I get too full, the heartburn never comes."

"Oh, that would truly be a wonderful 'side-effect.'"

"I just try to relax and enjoy my food no matter what I eat."

CHAPTER 7

"What if I can't eat soon enough," I asked. "Like if I'm stuck in a meeting or something like that."

"Well for me, even if I've somehow allowed myself to get to the point where I'm starving, I can't use that as an excuse to pig out. I just have to force myself to eat slowly."

"I see."

"But I always do my best to keep from getting to that point," she continued. "Each step is so important. You can't leave out a single one, or you'll run the risk of gaining instead of losing, as you saw before. For instance, if you eat what you want and don't chew slowly and don't stop when you start to feel full, you could take in a lot more calories than you currently are, and that would be devastating. If you don't savor the taste, you won't have that satisfied feeling, and if you let yourself get too hungry, you will inevitably gorge yourself."

"Like I did today," I said.

"Well, what all did you have to eat this morning?" she asked.

"Nothing," I said. "That's the problem. I saved my appetite in anticipation of coming here."

"Oh, no, that's never good."

"I totally ignored step number five, 'Never let yourself get too hungry.' So, about how often do you eat, then?"

"Well there's no set rule, but I usually eat something probably about every couple of hours or so."

"You mean literally every two hours? I'd be huge if I did that."

"Well, I didn't say I eat a meal every couple of hours, now. Nowhere near that. But I do try to eat a little something about every two hours."

I sipped my now-cold coffee. "Some people say, 'Eat six small meals a day,' but I've never actually tried that."

"I've heard that, too," she said. "And the way I eat, it probably does work out to about six or seven times a day. Not meals, mind you. You know, I might grab a handful of nuts and eat them one by one. Or a couple of Oreos and milk."

"Oh my God," I said, "I love Oreos. I'm sure you eat the 'Double Stuf.'"

She nodded. "Absolutely. But I take the top cookie off and throw it away. I only end up eating the bottom cookie and the 'Stuf.'"

"Why doesn't that surprise me?"

"Well, they just taste better that way. To me, anyway. And as always, I eat them…"

We both said, "in moderation," at the same time, laughing.

"Of course, I usually eat the whole bag at one sitting," I confessed. It was an exaggeration, but not much of one.

"Ha!" she said, smiling. "I know you're joking. But then again, you know, I might grab a handful of raisons or granola or something equally healthy. Or then again, a few Cheetos and some Coke over ice. Whatever I'm in the mood for. Maybe a glass of smooth chardonnay and a slice of cheddar cheese."

"So, not even alcohol is off-limits?"

"No—with as much stress as I'm under at work?"

"Oh, me too," I said. "But that's the one thing I've always done 'in moderation.'"

"So have I, really. Well, since my college days, at any rate."

"Yeah," I said, smiling. "I may have overindulged a time or two back then, too."

Tom suddenly seemed to appear from nowhere. "How about another cup of coffee," he asked us both while tidying up the table.

Amanda had only taken a few sips from hers, both cups, and now I heard her say, "Just one more."

I wasn't complaining. I was glad she wasn't in any hurry to leave. I had managed to drink both of my cups dry, however. "One more for me too, then," I said.

He looked down at me. "And have you changed your mind about dessert?" he asked cheerfully.

I was oh, so full by now, but I was definitely craving something sweet. "Oh, I don't know if I should," I said.

He smiled. "Well, let me see if I can entice you," he said. "Today we have a wonderfully rich crème brulée made with real vanilla beans and demerara sugar. And we also have our amazing bread pudding with a creamy New Orleans rum sauce." He looked at Amanda, his smile reaching his eyes. "And of course, we have our famous homemade turtle cheesecake, your favorite."

"That is my favorite," she agreed, nodding. "I think I'll have that, Tom. But I'll probably be taking most of it with me."

"Of course," he said, "that's no problem." Then looking back at me, he continued, "We also have our delicious tiramisu with creamy mascarpone cheese and Kahlua, topped off with an exquisite imported chocolate. Our from-scratch banana cream pie piled high with a fluffy, home-made double-whipped meringue…"

I had decided to do as I was pretty sure she was going to do—taste a bite or two now and take the rest with me for later. Would I be sitting at home this evening craving the tiramisu? I loved tiramisu. "I'll have the tiramisu," I blurted.

He smiled. "You won't be disappointed," he said. "It's delicious."

I looked at Amanda, but continued speaking to Tom, "I'll be taking most of mine home, as well."

"Yes," he said, "that might be a good idea. It's very rich, you know. I'll be right out with your desserts and fresh coffee then."

She looked at me. "I think you're getting the hang of it."

"Oh, I think I am, too," I said. "It's great. Please don't stop. You were telling me how you normally eat…So, you rarely ever sit down and eat a meal like we are today?"

"Oh, no, I do this quite often," she said. "But if I eat a 'meal,' I only eat parts of it, as I did today. Remember it's quantity not quality that gets you."

"Quantity not quality?"

"Yes, it's not what you eat that makes you gain weight, it's how much you eat. It's not what you eat, it's how you eat it."

"I see," I said.

Tom was suddenly back with our desserts. He'd brought each of us a perfectly sized dessert to-go box along with.

The tiramisu looked even more wonderful than he had described it—the bottom layer of Kahlua-soaked lady fingers, then a layer of rich looking custard, then the fluffy layer of cream, and then it started over again—topped off with a whisper of chocolate shavings. As miserable as I was, I knew I wouldn't leave here without at least a taste. I had already blown it today, but I would definitely start my new way of eating tomorrow.

"Right now I feel that if I never eat another bite, it will be too soon," I said when he'd gone. "But I knew I would get home and wish I had gotten the dessert."

"And then you'd be craving it and looking for a substitute," she said.

"So, should I take just a small taste now, and maybe sometime after that miserable feeling goes away, maybe take a couple of more bites?"

She nodded, her fork already in hand. "And really savor the taste of it. Truly enjoy it as never before. And then even later, maybe have a couple of more bites. And maybe have some again tomorrow."

"That's exactly what I'm going to do," I said. "I'm going to make it last as long as I possibly can."

"With something as rich as dessert, I normally take even smaller bites," she said, carving out the tiniest sliver of her cheesecake—smaller than a dime, even. I did the same with the tiramisu, although mine wasn't quite as small as hers. Oh, well, I was still new at this. Not that I wasn't capable of carving out a small bite, it was just that I had been carving extra-large bites for some forty-something years. Old habits are hard to break. I could see this was definitely going to take some practice.

We both sat there, taking our time luxuriating in the flavor. It had to be the absolute best tiramisu to ever graze the surface of my tongue. Or maybe it just seemed that way because it was the first time I had ever really, thoroughly tasted it.

When we'd both swallowed all traces of our bites, she said, "But going back to what we were talking about earlier—eating a little throughout the day. When I was in high school, there was this really cute guy who moved in across the street from us, and I was really surprised when he asked me out because I was a very unattractive teenager."

I found that very hard to believe. "I can't imagine that."

"Trust me," she said. "Braces and everything. Anyway, we dated for a while, and he was a few years older than I was, and he ended up joining the Navy. We sort of lost touch for a while, and then I saw him one day while he was on leave. He had joined the Navy as a 'skinny teenager,' and now he had really filled out—almost chubby. He even had a little pot belly and he was only about twenty or twenty-one."

She paused for a moment, sliding the rest of her piece of turtle cheesecake into the to-go box and fastening the lid.

"We were standing out on his front lawn," she continued, "or his parents' front lawn, talking. And he patted his stomach and mentioned having gained weight. And I told him I was surprised because I would've thought he would have lost weight instead of gaining. I said, 'I thought they really worked you hard in the military.' And he said, 'No, that's only in basic training.' He said he had gained weight because he was eating three square meals a day. And I thought he was crazy because I had always been taught that it was eating between meals that made you gain weight."

"That's what I always thought, too," I said. It was all I could do to do as she had done and put the dessert into the to-go box, but I somehow forced myself. I could hardly wait until that miserable, stuffed feeling went away so I could have some more.

"But in reality," she continued, "he had been eating haphazardly all his life, only eating when he wanted something to eat, on his own schedule, not anyone else's. Now he had to eat at a specific time and eat a lot so as not to get hungry before the next meal-time."

"So, it was as you said, eating so much at one time that made him gain?"

"Yes," she said, "I think so. You asked how I got started with this...I think my past experiences kind of stayed in the back of my mind and then, when I started college, I began to gain weight. You know...the old 'Freshman 15,' as they say."

"Yes, I guess it comes from being away from home, eating three full meals in the cafeteria."

"I think that's exactly it," she said. "But I decided to try what I'd seen other people do over the years. I'd watched people eat for some time by then. So, one summer, between semesters, I started eating slowly and eating about half the amount I would normally eat—I guess subconsciously following these five steps. And before I knew it, I had lost two sizes. A lot more than I had even initially gained. I was actually too thin and had to gain some of it back."

"Wow! I'd love to have that problem."

She had only eaten part of her "borrowed" appetizer, eaten mostly just the toppings off her salad, less than half of her entrée, and drunk only a few sips from her Sprite. I, on the other hand, had eaten almost all of my entrée, all of my salad, all but the one appetizer I had given her, and several bites of her meal, as well. Plus, the tiny bite of the tiramisu. I was starving when I arrived...and completely miserable now.

"You know, I really hate that stuffed, miserable feeling," I said. "But I always seem to end up with it...like now."

"Oh, I know exactly what you mean. Most people feel guilty about what they eat. How much fat or sugar or calories it has. Instead, I feel guilty when I eat too fast and overeat. I feel guilty about how much I eat rather than what I eat. Especially when I eat too much at one time. If I had ordered the appetizer, I probably wouldn't have ordered anything else."

"You mean you would have ordered the appetizer for your meal and nothing else? You really weren't kidding when you said 'anything goes.'"

She nodded. "Or I might have eaten the appetizer and a few bites of the entrée here, then gotten a to-go box and taken the rest home and 'grazed' on it the remainder of the day and probably even had some left for tomorrow."

"This is really a whole new way of looking at things for me," I said.

"Well, I certainly can't guarantee you'll lose weight," she said. "But I know there are times in my life when I'm very stressed and I forget to follow these steps. I start eating while I'm worrying about something—whether it be my job or my kids or whatever. I forget to relax and eat slowly and taste my food, and then I overindulge. And if I continue to do it, I find myself starting to gain."

"That stands to reason," I said.

"I have to regroup," she continued. "Unwind. Tell myself that nothing is worth putting on weight that will make my worst problems even worse. I go back to basics. These five simple steps that I had never verbalized until I began talking with you."

"I'm just so grateful I was the one you chose to share it all with."

CHAPTER 8

I hadn't seen her in well over a month. About a week after our lunch engagement, she had been called away on assignment to help finish setting up our new office in Charlotte.

She was pouring herself a cup of coffee when I entered the break room. "Michelle!" she squealed. "I was just about to come by your office." She reached out to hug me.

"Oh, Amanda, I'm so glad you're back," I said, wrapping my arms around her.

"Wow," she said, stepping back and eyeing me up and down. "You're looking great already."

"Thanks!"

"What's it been, only a month?"

"Maybe a little over," I said, silently beaming inside.

"I see you're not wearing a jacket."

"Yeah," I said, nodding. I wanted to twirl around and show her how much smaller my rear-end looked, but I had a while to go before I would be that confident. "No jacket anymore. I just started that this week, as a matter of fact. And I owe it all to you."

"No, no," she said, "you deserve all the credit."

"It's been hard giving it up—like giving up a security blanket."

"Oh, I definitely think you're ready," she said, still eyeing me. "How much have you lost?"

"I'm not sure about the weight," I said, "but I've definitely lost at least one dress size."

"That's terrific!"

"I'm not exactly ready to try blue jeans yet, but hopefully soon."

"Oh, I'm sure it won't be long." She picked up her cup. "Pour yourself some coffee. Do you have time to sit down?"

"Sure," I said, pulling an insulated paper cup from the top of the stack. I added a squirt of hazelnut creamer.

When I joined her at our same table, she said, "So, how's Jennifer doing?"

"Well, not great yet," I admitted, sitting down across from her, "but I think she's actually doing a little better."

"So, they still haven't gotten back together?"

"No, and I'm afraid she's still heartsick. I told you she'd been calling him, crying all the time, begging him to come back to her?"

"No, I hadn't heard that," she said. "That's not good."

"I know…it was disgusting. I finally told her he was never going to come back to her as long as she was acting like that. I mean, who wants to be with a basket case? I asked her if she would want to be with somebody who was acting like she was—if she had broken up with a guy and he was crying all the time, throwing himself at her, following her around like a puppy. I told her she needed to start acting like the girl he fell in love with and then, if he still didn't come back, she would at least maintain her dignity." I sipped my coffee. "I really think it's a little too late for her dignity, but I didn't tell her that."

"That's good advice," she said. "Did she take it?"

I nodded. "Surprisingly enough, she did. I was shocked."

"And is it working?" she asked.

"Well, he actually did call her the other day."

"Really? That's great!"

"She finally stopped calling him and sure enough, he broke down and called her. You know how it is when you think someone is getting over you."

"Yeah, it seems people want most what they can't have."

"Just like with food," I said unable to resist the parallel.

"It's human nature," she agreed, nodding. "So, the tables have taken another turn, then."

"And she actually kept her cool," I said. "I was listening to her on the phone, but she didn't know it. Then, when she hung up, she told me he said he was going to stop seeing the other girl—that he never really cared for her at all."

"Just as you thought."

"Right," I said. "He was just so upset that he was trying anything he could to get over her."

"So, they're getting back together, then?"

"Well no, he didn't say he was ready for that yet. And he'd be a fool to just turn around and take her back. But she says she's going to get back to her old self with or without him."

"I think that's the healthiest thing she can do," she said.

"Yes, I feel much better about it, now. And maybe she actually will get to the point where she can be okay without him. But I think she really is in love with him."

"Well, I certainly hope everything works out for her," she said sincerely.

"Yeah, if it's meant to be, I'm sure it will be." My coffee had gotten cold and I had only taken a few sips. And I had forgotten to "savor the flavor." Thank goodness I hadn't drunk too much and wasted all those hazelnut calories. "Can I get you a refill?" I asked her, standing.

"Yes, please—just a little."

"Hazelnut?" I emptied both of our cups into the sink and refilled them from a fresh pot that someone else had made.

"Yes," she said. "I usually wait until afternoon to start on the flavored stuff, but this is close enough."

I usually waited until afternoon, as well. Regular coffee just seemed to feel better in the mornings. I knew artificial creamers weren't exactly good for you, but I had also taken up her habit of only taking a few sips from every cup I drank.

"The 'mother's dress' is still on hold, then?" she asked when I returned to the table.

"For now, yes," I said. "In fact, I've put off buying any new clothes at all for a while." I gestured toward my outfit. "This is from about five years ago when I went on what was, hopefully, my last fad diet—when I lost a lot of weight, only to gain it all back again. I want to lose that other size before I actually spend any money. That will be two full dress sizes."

"That's fantastic!"

I sat back down. "I can't possibly thank you enough, Amanda. I still have more to go, but I'm ecstatic about it."

"Oh, I was very happy to do what I could," she said.

I asked her how the Charlotte setup had gone and she told me it had been hectic, but a success. Then she asked me about the kinds of things I had been eating.

"Well, I'm eating only the stuff I like and want," I explained, "just as you advised. In the morning, I might eat cereal, I might eat part of an omelet, or I might eat leftover pizza from the night before. It's great. I don't obsess over it. I don't feel guilty about it...that is, unless I eat too much of it. I no longer feel guilty or obsess about how many calories or carbs or fat something has. It's all about quantity, now. All about moderation—I do my best not to eat very much of anything, especially at one time."

"And don't you find that regulating the quantity is much easier than trying to stay away from foods everyone around you is eating? Foods you crave and love?"

"Much easier." I sipped my hazelnut coffee—and savored it this time. "I can eat the same foods other people do, I just eat those foods a lot more slowly and taste them a lot more fully and enjoy them a lot more than I used to."

"That's great," she said.

"I've been breaking the rules," I said. "Like you, I've never cared for the crust on bread, but I never thought to peel it off. I just went ahead and ate it anyway. Now I peel it off, especially on sandwiches, and eat only the good stuff."

She was smiling. "Like you said, 'It's a whole new way of looking at things.'"

"It really is," I agreed. "I only like the topping of pizza, too, so I leave the crust just as you do."

"And do you still save the best for last?" she asked.

"Oh, no, never," I said. "The other day I had a vegetable plate from O'Malley's down the street. I love their creamed corn, and normally I would scarf down all the other veggies and my bread and save the corn for last. I'd be miserable before I even took my first bite of it. Not anymore. Now I eat most of the corn first and just a couple of bites of everything else for balance. And I try to leave a bite or two of the corn, also. I really had to practice that—leaving something on my plate—but it really helps to say, 'This is going to be my last bite,' like you suggested. And usually before I get to that point—when I think it's getting close to time to stop—I start taking even smaller and smaller bites to make it last even longer."

"That's a great idea," she said. "I'll have to try that."

"I mean, what are the chances that I'm going to magically have the exact amount on my plate that I need to be full? And I think it's better to assume that there's too much than too little. I'm like you, I hate to throw food away, so I try all the alternatives—eat it later, save it for the kids, get a to-go box."

She sipped her coffee. "And of course, you can always do the split-diet thing—if you know you can't take it with you, talk the other person into splitting the entrée with you. But then you might have to compromise on what you want when you order, and that's never a good thing."

I was thoughtful for a moment. "It's sad to say, but no matter how much you leave on your plate, you're not going to help starving children. It's better to simply take out less or ask for smaller servings. And you're not really wasting money if you don't eat everything on your plate."

She shook her head. "Like you said, it ends up costing you more trying to get rid of it later."

"And most people waste much more money on diets—like diet books, mail-order food, diet milkshakes, specialty foods, treadmills, bikes, clothes from gaining and losing, the list goes on."

She nodded. "There will be times when you just have to leave what's leftover."

"You're right," I said. "And for that reason, I almost never go to all-you-can-eat buffets anymore—which Bill wasn't too crazy about at first. But then he saw how much weight I was losing and decided to try the diet with me."

"That's great," she said.

"Of course, he's a man—he's lost a lot more than I have." I smiled. "But then again, he had a lot more to lose."

She laughed. "But it really sounds like you're following the steps pretty closely."

I nodded. "I think I am. I'm taking small bites, about the size of a nickel or smaller—depending on what I'm eating—and chewing them slowly, and you were right, I do get full with a lot less food."

"That's a good rule of thumb," she said.

"And if I do have to eat something that I'm really not that crazy about, just to keep from getting too hungry, I force myself to take small bites and chew slowly, as you advised. Like if I somehow end up at a restaurant I'm not particularly fond of. Or if I'm invited to someone's home for dinner and they aren't serving anything I really like, I eat as little as possible without offending them."

"Yeah, I've always found that to be a tricky situation."

"And the lack of taste makes it difficult to 'savor the flavor.'"

"Yes, it does," she agreed. "And how is that working out for you—savoring the flavor?"

"Oh, that's the best part," I said. "I'm really trying to concentrate on how amazing everything tastes—down to the last morsel." I'd had to admit to myself that I had never taken the time to actually taste my food. I was always trying to finish the current bite so I could hurry and get the next one into my mouth. Now I was trying to make each bite last as long as I possibly could.

"That's exactly what I do," she said. "Isn't it wonderful?"

"It is. And the flavor! Oh my God. I really never knew what I was missing by wolfing down my food—probably only tasting the first couple of bites—then thinking about something else while the rest of my meal went down, unnoticed."

She was nodding. "Believe it or not, there have been times when I've even had to remind myself to concentrate on the flavor of chocolate."

"Oh, me too. But I'm not as obsessed with it now. As with the Reese's, I used to crave things and drive myself crazy trying to avoid them and generally end up eating them in the end anyway. Now, I know they're there and I can have some or anything else I might happen to want. It's a great feeling."

"I know exactly what you mean. It's just so hard to keep from eating something once you start craving it or when someone else is eating it in front of you."

"It really is," I said. "And I did as you suggested—practiced leaving something for later. And then I started taking out smaller amounts and still leaving something every time. And you were right, as long as I know I can have a little more later, it makes it easier to stop eating something that I'm really enjoying. If I eat it all now, it will all be gone, and that makes me want to leave some for the next time."

"And do you do like I do?" she asked. "Say, 'this is my last bite,' a couple of times before it really is your last bite?"

"Yes, I do," I said, nodding. "I liked your analogy about the smoker needing that last cigarette for closure. That's exactly what it's like for me. But sometimes I end up taking a couple of more bites anyway, as you said."

"And that's okay, occasionally," she admitted.

"But those extra last bites are becoming fewer and further between. And the taste is always at the forefront of my mind, even if someone is sitting across the table from me, talking. Even if it's something I'm interested in, I'm constantly thinking about the taste."

"That really takes practice, too," she said.

"It really does," I agreed. I was struggling to do it now—taste my coffee while I talked to her.

"And can you tell you're eating less now, quantity-wise?"

"Oh, yes, absolutely. I'm eating a lot less, and now it's stretched out over the whole day. I used to eat two huge meals a day. I'd skip breakfast, of course, because it was the easiest to skip. I'm usually not hungry early in the morning. But then by lunch-time I'd be starving, and I would eat about twice as much as I really needed. And I usually tried to eat diet foods at lunch, but obviously that didn't do any good."

"Diet foods have never worked for me," she said. "They've always left me wanting something else."

"Oh, me too," I said. I took a sip from my coffee and savored it. "And then dinner has always been a family thing, and I'd be tired, and talking to Bill and the kids about all our days and homework and such, just raking in the food, going back for seconds. And then I'd be so miserable I'd have to change into sweatpants."

She nodded and said, "Yes, I know a lot of people who do that."

"I've stopped all that now," I happily said. "It's just ridiculous when you think about it. Eating a huge plate of food simply because it was in front of me. I would eat so much and so fast—usually even going back for more. And then, of course, I'd have indigestion all night long."

"Bless your heart," she said. "How's that going now?"

"Oh, I almost never get it anymore. Now the only time I get it is if, for some reason, I've overeaten or if I've eaten too fast. And I almost never do that anymore. Only a few times that I've been stressed and had too much going on to concentrate on the five steps."

"It's definitely never a good thing to eat when you're stressed out," she said. "I know I eat much more than I intend to. I have to force myself to clear my mind before I eat."

"Me too!"

"So, about how often are you eating now?"

"I'm pretty much doing as you suggested, eating about every two hours—just a few bites of something."

"That's good," she said. "So, you're eating breakfast everyday now?"

I nodded. "Even if I'm not really hungry, I find that if I eat just a little something, I eat a lot less the rest of the day."

"I almost never skip breakfast," she told me. "Literally, only when I'm going to the doctor for tests or something. I usually eat something within an hour or so after I wake up."

"So do I, now," I said. "And dinner is still a family thing, but now I probably eat less than half of what I used to eat during the time it takes them to eat their normal amount. Sometimes I may not be full when I stop, but if I wait a few minutes, it catches up with me. And then I actually don't want to eat any more."

"That works for me, too. I usually have to do that—stop and let it catch up—if I've let myself get a little too hungry."

I nodded. "Especially then. I usually eat three so-called 'meals' a day. That is, I eat something around meal times. That way I can eat while other people are eating. I just try to eat slowly enough that I've eaten a lot less than they have when we're all finished. And it's usually balanced. Sometimes at work, I may just snack all day. I might get a little something from the cafeteria or get one of those great cinnamon rolls from the kiosk downstairs and only eat the center, as you do. Or if I want something healthy, I go to the little shop on the corner and get some fresh fruit or something. But even when I eat healthy, I always make sure I follow the steps. It has to be something I really love and something I'm in the mood for. Like those toasted walnuts they have."

"Aren't those divine?"

"Oh, they're flawless. And I usually have some left over for a snack later."

"Oh, me too, always." About that time, we heard someone paging her on the overhead speaker. "Well, I guess I'd better be getting back to my office." She scooted her chair back and said, "You don't know how glad I am that everything is working out so well for you, Michelle."

"And you don't know how grateful I am to you, for everything."

CHAPTER 9

I was embarrassed to just now be returning them—her scissors. Justin had long ago finished his science project, and we had gotten a very acceptable B plus. Not bad considering neither of us knew anything about $E=mc2$ before we started. We had created a model that explained how Einstein's equation had been applied to the making of the first atomic bomb. The research had been very interesting. Unfortunately, I had been the one to undertake it all, and I had a feeling my son still didn't even know so much as what a neutron was, much less the part it played in the splitting of the atom.

I was sitting in the chair in front of her desk when she returned from the break room that afternoon carrying two cups of coffee. She had been heading that way just as I was about to knock and had offered to bring me a cup. And now the delectable aroma of the hazelnut creamer entered the room before she did, and I was thrilled to know that, not only was it in her cup, it was in mine, as well.

Yes, I had officially gone back to flavored creamers…in moderation, of course. I didn't necessarily add them every day, and usually only in the afternoons. And I was taking smaller sips and drinking less coffee in the long run—reheating it whenever it got too cool or pouring it out and starting over.

"I got my invitation to the wedding," she said, handing me my cup. "It's still good, right? Same time, same location?"

"Yes, everything's back on exactly as it was. Things couldn't be better."

"That's fantastic," she said, rolling her chair from behind her desk to sit adjacent to me. "I'm definitely planning on being there."

"Great! I was so hoping you'd be able to make it."

"Well, even though I've never met her, I feel as if I know her. I was so glad when you called and told me they had worked things out."

I turned my chair more to face her. "As soon as she started acting like her old self, there he was again, back on bended knee."

"And you look absolutely amazing," she said sincerely. "I can't wait to see you in the 'mother's dress.'"

"Well, I've tried it on, and it actually does look pretty good."

"I'll bet it looks great. And you certainly pass the blue jeans test now. Hands down."

Those of us who didn't deal directly with customers were allowed to wear jeans on Fridays. I hadn't even realized she had looked at me as I passed her in the doorway. "You noticed?"

"Absolutely," she said. "You probably turn heads all the time now."

"Well, I wouldn't go that far," I said. "But everyone I know seems to notice I've lost weight. Of course they all wanted to know how I did it. Do you mind if I share with my friends and family?"

"Oh, no, of course not. I think it's great."

"I was hoping you would say that because I sort of already did. My sister absolutely adores me now."

She smiled. "I'm fortunate enough to have a job where I can eat whenever I want and so are you. We can snack at our desks just about any time or get up and go to the break room at any given moment. We have a lot of freedom. But even if we didn't, you know, most people get a break every couple of hours anyway, so it shouldn't be too much of a problem for anybody to follow."

"Oh, I agree. There's just no way I can thank you enough for everything, Amanda. I owe you so much."

"Not at all," she said, waving me off. "I'm just glad to see it work for somebody else. For as long as I can remember, people have said things like, 'I don't know how you stay so thin, every time I see you, you're eating.' Or they've asked me, 'How do you stay so thin when you eat all the time?' They assumed because I was eating all the time that I ate a lot. But as I said, it's not what you eat, it's how much you eat. It's not quality, it's quantity. And some people will probably say, 'Well, I can just starve myself and eat one meal a day and get a lot less calories than you do.' But for some reason, it doesn't seem to work that way."

"No," I said, "everyone I've ever heard say they eat one meal a day is usually overweight. And besides, why would you want to eat one meal a day when you can eat a little all day long? And eat what you want? Not tasteless diet stuff, but things your body is telling you to eat. Things you love and crave."

She was nodding. "And like I said, there'll be times when you might get off track—there are times when I do. It takes a while to make it a habit, a new way of life, second nature."

"It really does," I said. "Sometimes I'll be halfway through my meal and realize I haven't even tasted it. Even if it's been something I've been craving. And I just have to tell myself to slow down. Tune everything else out. Taste every bite thoroughly."

"I know exactly what you mean. I still do the same thing."

"And then there will be other times when I have a lot on my mind or I'm rushed because of a deadline and a couple of days later, I'll get on the scale and realized I've started to gain. Then I have to remind myself of the five steps, get myself back on track, forget about work and everything else while I'm eating. That's my time. And a couple of days later, my weight is back to where it was. I just have to remind myself not to get so caught up in everyday stress and pressures that my diet suffers."

"I still have to work on that, too," she admitted.

"But knowing this is all I have to do? That I don't have to give up chocolate or fried chicken or yeast rolls or anything else I love. All I have to do is not eat very much of it, eat it slowly, and thoroughly enjoy it? Just knowing that makes me know this is something I can do forever."

"Oh, I'm sure you can," she said.

"You know, I didn't realize it, but I had actually been taking in a lot more calories eating diet foods that I didn't like than I am now—eating all the things I do like. Probably because I would usually end up eating a lot more, trying to satisfy whatever craving I happened to be having at the time."

"And you probably felt full but never satisfied."

"Oh, without a doubt," I said. "And this is not like any other diet I've tried. I mean, you can go to any restaurant, any party. You don't have to bring your own food, wait for it in the mail, worry about how many points it's worth. You just have to listen to your body—pay attention to what you're eating. Yeah, you may start to get hungry again in a couple of hours, but you need to eat again in a couple of hours anyway."

"That's right," she agreed, nodding.

I knew I needed to be getting back to my desk but I wasn't quite ready. "And now that I've lost my weight, I'm going to try exercising more," I told her. "I've been walking a little every day, but that's something I've been doing all along, even before this. But now I'm walking longer distances. And something I never did was take the stairs. Lately, I've been scaling the three flights to get to my office every morning and taking them again anytime I need to go downstairs for anything during the day. I've also been parking away from the building like you do. I haven't tackled push-mowing the lawn yet, but I'm willing to give it a try."

She laughed. "Now, when I said I did my own yard work, I neglected to tell you that I have a small yard."

"Yeah, I may be getting a little too ambitious. Mine is pretty big. Maybe I'll just use that gym membership I've been paying for all these years."

"That might be a good idea, then," she said.

"I think I really need to tone up. But you know, what's wonderful about this is that I no longer have to worry about regaining my weight. I know that if I gain weight, it's not because of what I eat, it's because of how much I eat. And if I start to lose too much, all I have to do is eat a little more. It all seems to be about balance."

"You are exactly right," she said.

"This has been the easiest diet I've ever been on. I haven't even been remotely tempted to go back to my old way of doing things. It has required some practice—practice leaving something on my plate, practice listening to my body, practice chewing slowly and tuning everything else out and concentrating on the flavor. But it's been great. Like you said, a whole new way of eating."

"Yes, it really is."

I knew I was staying away from my desk too long. "I guess I'd better be getting back to work," I said, standing.

She rose to walk me to the door. "Well, if I don't see you before, I guess I'll see you at the wedding. I can hardly wait. I'm sure it's going to be beautiful."

At that moment I knew that, not only had I gained a new way of life, I had also gained a life-long friend. "I'm so glad you're going to be there," I said.

I had changed my life and it was all because of her four simple words: "In All Things, Moderation."

And those five common-sense steps:

1 - Eat what you want and only what you want
2 - Take small bites and chew them slowly
3 - Savor the flavor
4 - Never let yourself get too full
5 - Never let yourself get too hungry

"By the way," she said, smiling as we reached the door, "there's turtle cheesecake in the break room."

And I did stop by the break room on my way back to my office. And I did get a piece of turtle cheesecake. But this time, I only got one piece. And this time, I wasn't licking my fork clean when I made it to the door.